MIGRAINES

UNDERSTANDING HOW MIGRAINES OCCUR
AND POSSIBLE WAYS OF HEALING IT

DR. A. RAMOS

Contents

INTRODUCTION

Beyond just being excruciating headaches, migraines are intricate neurological events marked by excruciating, throbbing pain that is frequently accompanied by additional symptoms. These episodes can cause discomfort and disturbance to daily living, which can have a considerable impact. Studying migraines' unique characteristics, causes, and manifestation patterns is essential to understanding them. Let's investigate the realm of migraines and the difficulties that sufferers face.

CHAPTER ONE

A Definition of Migraines

Recurrent, severe headaches that are usually accompanied by additional symptoms are the hallmark of the headache illness known as migraines. These headaches are typically confined to one side of the head and frequently have a throbbing or pulsating quality. A person's everyday life can be greatly impacted by migraines, which can linger for hours or even days.

Pain Level:

It is well known that migraines can cause moderate to severe discomfort. Common descriptions of the pain include pulsing or throbbing, and regular physical activity may make it worse.

One-sided Position:

Although they can impact one or both sides of the brain, migraines typically present as unilateral, or one-sided. During different instances, the discomfort may alternate across sides.

Extra Symptoms:

Headache is not the only symptom associated with migraines. These can include light or sound sensitivity (phonophobia), nausea, vomiting, and photophobia.

Aura

Before or during the headache phase, some people report experiencing an aura, which is a visual or sensory sensation. Auras can cause sensory abnormalities like tingling in the hands or face, or they can cause visual disruptions like flashing lights or zigzag lines.

Time:

The length of migraines varies. They can be categorized as chronic (occurring 15 days or more per month for at least three months) or episodic (occurring less than 15 days per month).

Triggers:

Numerous things, such as particular diets, stress, hormonal fluctuations, sleep deprivation, and environmental variables, can cause migraines.

It's crucial to remember that not everyone experiences migraines in the same way, and that not all migraines have an aura. Individual differences exist in the frequency, severity, and precise symptoms experienced by each person. The quality of life can be significantly impacted by migraines, as they might cause missed work or social events when they occur.

Finding triggers for migraines, changing one's lifestyle, and occasionally using medicine to reduce symptoms are all part of the diagnosis and treatment process. It is imperative that people with migraines seek medical attention in order to have a precise diagnosis and individualized treatment plan.

Reasons and Initiators

Although the precise etiology of migraines is unknown, a combination of neurological, environmental, and hereditary factors are thought to be involved. Many times, particular triggers that differ from person to person cause migraines. Determining the sources of migraines can be essential to controlling and averting attacks. The following are typical migraine triggers and causes:

1. Genetic Elements:

The chance of having migraines is increased in families where migraines are present. Migraine susceptibility may be influenced by specific hereditary variables.

2. Changes in the Neurology:

Abnormal brain activity, namely involving the trigeminal nerve and its branches, has been linked to migraines. Pain and other symptoms are brought on by the production of inflammatory chemicals and neurotransmitters as a result.

3. Changes in Hormones:

Migraines can be brought on by changes in hormones, particularly in women. Migraines associated with the menstrual cycle, pregnancy, or menopause affect a lot of women.

4. Antagonists in the surroundings:

Migraines can be brought on by specific environmental variables. Among them are:

Sensual stimuli include intense noises, bright lights, and powerful smells.

Weather variations: shifts in the barometric pressure, excessive humidity, or sharp temperature swings.

Altitude changes: Some people get migraines when they travel to high elevations.

5. Sleep disturbances:

Migraines can be brought on by irregular sleep patterns, sleep deprivation, or adjustments to sleep schedules.

6. Nutritional Elements:

Some people are known to be migraine triggers for particular foods and drinks. Typical offenders consist of:

Caffeine (withdrawal that is abrupt or extreme).

cheeses that have aged.

processed meals with MSG (monosodium glutamate) or other additives.

Alcohol particularly red wine.

Cocoa.

7. Dehydration:

Migraine onset may be influenced by dehydration and inadequate fluid consumption.

8. Stress

Many migraine sufferers find that emotional stress and anxiety are important triggers. Migraine prevention may be aided by stress-reduction methods, such relaxation training.

9. Overuse of Medication:

Medication-overuse headaches, which can worsen migraines, can result from the regular use of some drugs, such as painkillers or medications designed specifically to treat migraines.

10. Factors related to the body:

Some people experience migraines when they expend a lot of energy or suddenly move physically.

It's crucial to remember that different people have quite different triggers, and what causes migraines in one person might not in another. Working with a healthcare professional and keeping a migraine journal can help you see trends and create specialized migraine management plans. Individual needs may dictate the recommendation of preventive drugs, stress reduction strategies, and lifestyle modifications.

Beyond just headaches, a variety of symptoms are associated with migraines. The several phases of a migraine episode and the fluctuating nature of the symptoms add to the intricacy of this neurological disorder. Let's examine the typical phases and symptoms of a migraine:

Common Migraine Symptoms:

A throbbing headache

A migraine is characterized by a throbbing or pulsating headache. Often ranging from mild to severe, the pain can be made worse by regular physical exercise.

One-sided headache:

Although they can impact one or both sides of the brain, migraines typically present as unilateral, or one-sided. During different instances, the discomfort may alternate across sides.

Aura

Auras might appear before or during the headache phase in certain people. Usually, auras are visual disruptions like blind spots, zigzag lines, or flashing lights. Auras, however, can also cause changes in sensation, such as tingling in the hands or cheeks.

CHAPTER TWO

Vomiting and nauseous:

During an episode, a lot of people with migraines experience nausea and occasionally vomiting.

Light Sensitivity (Photophobia):

Light sensitivity is a typical side effect of migraines. Sunlight or bright lighting may make symptoms worse.

Phonophobia (sensitivity to sound):

Sound sensitivity is another common symptom. Certain sounds or loud noises might exacerbate the pain of a migraine.

Sensitivity to senses:

During a migraine attack, some people may become more sensitive to touch or particular textures.

Weakness and Fatigue:

Physically taxing migraines can cause weariness and a generalized weakness.

Having trouble concentrating:

One typical symptom is "migraine brain," which is defined as difficulty concentrating or feeling mentally foggy.

Vertigo or dizziness:

Some people may get vertigo, or the feeling that something is spinning, when they have a migraine.

A migraine's phases:

Phase of Prodrome:

This stage, which comes on days or hours before the headache, is marked by mild behavioral, emotional, or energetic changes. Cravings for food, increased thirst, or other warning indicators may occur in certain people.

Phase of Aura:

Not everyone who has a migraine feels an aura. If so, this stage is characterized by particular neurological symptoms including altered sensations or vision problems. Usually, auras endure anywhere from 20 to 60 minutes.

Phase of a headache:

The most noticeable and frequently most incapacitating stage is the headache phase. The symptoms that accompany a throbbing headache might linger for hours or even days.

Phase of Postdrome:

After the headache phase, people may go through a postdrome, sometimes known as a "migraine hangover," which is characterized by persistent symptoms like weariness, irritation, and a general feeling of malaise.

It's critical to understand that not everyone experiences all phases or symptoms of a migraine, and that individual differences might be significant. Every person's experience with migraines is different due to variations in the frequency, severity, and length of the condition. For a precise diagnosis and tailored treatment, seeking medical advice is essential for migraine sufferers.

Identification and Medical Assessment

A comprehensive assessment of symptoms, medical history, and, in certain situations, further testing to rule out other possible headache causes, are usually part of the diagnosis and medical evaluation of migraines. This is a summary of the procedure:

1. Health Background:

The medical professional will begin by obtaining a thorough medical history, which will include details regarding the frequency, severity, and nature of headaches. We'll talk about any related symptoms, causes, and family history of migraines.

2. Headache Journal:

Maintaining a headache journal that documents the onset, length, and features of headaches as well as possible triggers can be very helpful in determining the cause and developing a treatment strategy.

3. Physical Assessment:

One way to evaluate general health and rule out other possible headache reasons is to perform a physical checkup. It is also possible to do neurological exams to look for any anomalies.

4. Standards for Diagnosing Migraines:

If the symptoms are consistent with a migraine diagnosis, the medical professional will frequently make this determination using accepted diagnostic criteria. The International Classification of Headache Disorders (ICHD) lists common criteria.

5. Discard Any Further Circumstances:

It is necessary to rule out other possible causes of headaches and neurological symptoms in order to guarantee an accurate diagnosis. To screen for structural abnormalities or other medical issues, this may require imaging investigations like computed tomography (CT) scans or magnetic resonance imaging (MRI).

6. Evaluation of Aura:

The features and duration of any auras will be evaluated. This aids in separating aura-associated migraines from other kinds of headaches.

7. Lifestyle and Trigger Factors:

An important aspect of the evaluation is looking into possible triggers and lifestyle factors that could be associated with migraines. This entails evaluating food practices, stress levels, sleep patterns, and other possible environmental variables.

8. Laboratory Examinations:

For the most part, migraines can be diagnosed without the need for laboratory testing. They could be required, nevertheless, in order to rule out any additional medical issues that might be causing headaches.

9. Speaking with Experts:

A referral to a neurologist or headache specialist may be advised in certain situations, particularly if there are unusual characteristics or if the diagnosis is difficult.

10. Assessment of Effect on Everyday Life:

Determining how migraines affect daily activities, such as work, relationships, and general wellbeing, is essential to creating a successful treatment strategy.

Getting a precise diagnosis is essential to creating a customized migraine treatment plan. It enables medical professionals to customize interventions—such as acute care, preventive care, and lifestyle adjustments—to meet each patient's unique needs. People who are suffering from migraines are advised to speak with a medical expert for a thorough assessment and suitable treatment.

Methods of Therapy

Acute treatments to relieve symptoms during an episode, combined with lifestyle changes and preventive measures, are the methods used to treat migraines. Treatment for migraines is frequently customized according to the frequency, intensity, and unique features of the attacks. The following are typical methods of treating migraines:

1. Changes in Lifestyle:

Determine possible triggers and make lifestyle adjustments to address them. This could entail using relaxation techniques to manage stress, adhering to a regular sleep schedule, drinking plenty of water, and avoiding foods that are known to increase anxiety.

2. Drugs, Acute or Abortive:

The following drugs are taken during a migraine attack to reduce symptoms and shorten the length of the attack:

Pain relievers: Over-the-counter drugs such as aspirin, ibuprofen, or acetaminophen.

Triptans: Prescription drugs that restrict blood vessels and obstruct pain pathways to precisely target migraine symptoms.

3. Medications for prevention:

Preventive medicine may be provided to those who experience severe or regular migraines in order to lessen the frequency and intensity of episodes. These drugs could consist of:

Beta-blockers: Propranolol is one example.

Tricyclic antidepressants and selective serotonin reuptake inhibitors (SSRIs) are two types of antidepressants.

Drugs that prevent seizures: Topiramate and valproic acid, for example.

4. Biofeedback and Methods of Relaxation:

Stress management and migraine frequency can be decreased with the use of biofeedback and relaxation techniques such progressive muscle relaxation, guided visualization, and deep breathing.

5. Physical Medicine:

For many individuals, particularly those whose migraines are influenced by musculoskeletal issues, physical therapy could prove advantageous. Exercises, stretches, and massages are a few helpful techniques.

6. Therapy based on cognitive behavior (CBT):

Cognitive Behavioral Therapy (CBT) is a type of psychotherapy that can help control migraines by addressing stress, identifying triggers, and altering thought and behavior patterns associated with pain.

7. Hormone Treatment:

Hormone therapy or changing the way that they take contraceptives may be options for women whose migraines are linked to changes in their hormone levels.

8. Neuromodulation Tools:

Non-pharmacological methods of treating migraines may involve the use of devices like external trigeminal nerve stimulation (eTNS) or transcutaneous electrical nerve stimulation (TENS).

9. Botox injections:

A doctor may advise Botox injections for people who experience 15 or more headache days per month if they suffer from persistent migraines. To stop migraines, some muscles are injected with Botox.

10. Alternative Medical Interventions:

Alternative therapies like acupuncture, herbal supplements, or dietary adjustments help some people find comfort. It's crucial to go over these choices with a medical professional.

11. Modifications to Diet:

For some people, identifying and avoiding trigger foods as well as eating a balanced diet may help prevent migraines.

The distinctive needs, preferences, and reaction to interventions of each individual influence the choice of treatment. For migraine treatment to be effective, the patient and the healthcare professional must work together. For people who suffer from migraines, regular follow-up sessions and plan modifications may be required to maximize results and enhance quality of life.

Lifestyle Factors to Take Into Account

When it comes to controlling migraines and lessening the frequency and intensity of attacks, lifestyle factors are crucial. Changing one's lifestyle and forming healthy habits can enhance medical care and promote general wellbeing. The following are important lifestyle factors for people who suffer from migraines:

1. Preserve Consistent Sleeping Patterns:

Set and keep regular sleep schedules by going to bed and waking up at the same times each day. Aim for seven to nine hours of good sleep every night.

2. Control Your Stress:

Use stress-reduction strategies including yoga, mindfulness, meditation, and deep breathing. Migraine triggers can be avoided by locating and managing stressors.

3. Maintain Hydration:

Make sure you stay properly hydrated by consuming enough water throughout the day. For certain people, dehydration can be a migraine trigger.

4. Frequent Workout:

Regularly partake in mild physical activities, such cycling, swimming, or walking. Exercise can enhance general wellbeing and assist in lowering stress. It's crucial to refrain from engaging in strenuous or excessive physical activity when experiencing a migraine attack.

5. A well-rounded diet

Keep your diet well-balanced by eating regular meals and snacks. Determine which foods trigger migraines and stay away from them. Caffeine, alcohol, chocolate, and specific additives are a few typical foods that cause trigger reactions.

6. Limit your intake of coffee.

Pay attention to how much caffeine you consume. Caffeine can help some people with their migraines, but headaches can also be brought on by excessive or abrupt caffeine withdrawal. Continue consuming coffee at the same rate every day.

7. Create a Schedule:

Establish and follow a daily schedule that includes planned breaks, regular mealtimes, and sleep times. Having a routine can aid in regulating the body's internal clock.

8. Control Your Screen Time:

Limit the amount of time you spend using screens, especially bright-screened electronics. To lessen eye strain, take frequent breaks and think about using blue light filters.

9. Find and Steer Clear of Triggers:

Maintain a migraine journal to help you recognize and monitor possible triggers, such as particular meals, hormone fluctuations, or external circumstances. Once triggers have been identified, reduce exposure to them.

10. Methods of Relaxation:

Include relaxation methods like guided visualization, progressive muscle relaxation, and biofeedback in your everyday routine. These techniques can aid with tension and stress management.

11. Be Aware of Hormonal Shifts:

If hormonal fluctuations, such as those brought on by menstruation, are causing migraines for you, keep track of your periods and talk to a doctor about preventive treatments.

12. Sufficient Lighting

Make sure there is enough illumination in both your living and working areas. Steer clear of bright or flickering lights as these can give some people migraines.

13. Give Up Smoking:

If you smoke, think about giving it up. In addition to being harmful to one's overall health, smoking may also cause migraines in certain people.

14. Assist Mechanism:

Create a network of friends, family, or a medical professional to lean on for understanding, support, and guidance when things get hard.

Enhancing migraine management can be accomplished by combining medical therapies with a holistic approach that tackles lifestyle variables. Collaboration amongst healthcare practitioners is crucial in creating a customized strategy that caters to each patient's requirements and preferences. Long-term effectiveness in controlling this illness can be attributed to routine follow-up and candid discussion regarding lifestyle modifications and their effects on migraines.

Coping Mechanisms and Assistance

In addition to taking medication, managing migraines requires learning coping mechanisms, minimizing their influence on everyday activities, and asking for help when necessary. For those who are suffering from migraines, consider the following coping mechanisms and resources:

1. Knowledge and comprehension:

Find out more about migraines, including its causes, signs, and possible remedies. Having a thorough understanding of the illness enables people to make knowledgeable decisions about their care.

2. Record Your Migraines:

Keep a migraine journal to record the onset, length, and possible causes of your headaches. Patterns can be found and interactions with healthcare practitioners can be steered by this information.

3. Organize a Regular Schedule:

Establish a daily schedule that includes regular eating, sleeping, and rest periods.

CHAPTER THREE

Regularities that are predictable can assist lower stress and balance the body's internal clock.

4. Techniques for Stress Management:

Use stress-reduction strategies include progressive muscle relaxation, mindfulness, meditation, and deep breathing. Frequent practice can assist in reducing stress levels in general.

5. Recognize and Control Triggers:

Collaborate with medical professionals to recognize and control particular triggers. This could entail controlling hormone fluctuations, staying away from trigger foods, or taking care of environmental issues.

6. Plan of Acute Treatment:

Create an acute care plan after consulting a medical professional. Medications or techniques tailored to easing migraine symptoms may be part of this regimen.

7. Encouragement Setting:

Establish a welcoming atmosphere at work and home. Share information about your illness with your loved ones, friends, and coworkers so that they are aware of your needs while you are having migraine attacks.

8. Interact with Healthcare Professionals:

Keep lines of communication open with medical professionals. Talk about any concerns, therapy efficacy, or changes in symptoms. Scheduling routine follow-up visits can help to maximize care.

9. Participate in Support Groups:

Think about signing up for an online or in-person migraine support group. Making connections with people who have gone through comparable circumstances can offer insightful conversations, support, and a feeling of belonging.

10. Workplace Amenities:

If a migraine substantially affects one's ability to work, talk to your bosses about possible accommodations. This could involve modifying the work environment, offering remote work choices, or having flexible work hours.

11. Good Living Practices:

Make your general health a priority by forming a balanced diet, getting frequent exercise, and drinking enough water. These routines can improve general wellbeing.

12. Establish sensible objectives:

Set attainable objectives for your job, personal life, and everyday activities. During migraine episodes, acknowledge and accept your limitations and refrain from overexerting yourself.

13. Body-Mind Techniques:

Examine mind-body exercises like tai chi or yoga. These techniques can improve general wellbeing, stress relief, and relaxation.

14. Seek Expert Assistance:

Take into consideration contacting therapists, counselors, or psychologists for expert assistance. Other therapeutic modalities, such as cognitive-behavioral therapy (CBT), may be helpful in stress management and chronic condition management.

15. Adherence to Medication:

Comply with the recommended dosage schedule and the advice of your doctor for both acute and preventive care.

16. Sustain an optimistic attitude:

Pay attention to keeping an optimistic mindset. Even though migraines might be difficult, having a resilient outlook and appreciating little accomplishments can improve one's quality of life in general.

The best way for migraine sufferers to manage their illness may be to use a mix of these coping mechanisms and resources for assistance. Developing a thorough and long-lasting migraine care strategy requires personalizing strategies to each patient's preferences and requirements.

Preventive Actions

The goal of migraine preventive strategies is to lessen the frequency, intensity, and effects of migraine attacks. These methods frequently combine medication, lifestyle modifications, and other therapies. People who suffer from migraines may want to think about the following preventive measures:

1. Find and Steer Clear of Triggers:

Collaborate with medical professionals to pinpoint particular causes that lead to migraines. Some foods, hormone fluctuations, stress, and environmental conditions are common causes. Once triggers have been identified, reduce exposure to them.

2. Preserve Consistent Sleeping Patterns:

Make sure you go to bed and wake up at the same time every day to create consistent sleep patterns. It is essential to get enough good sleep if you want to avoid migraines.

3. Maintain Hydration:

Make sure you stay properly hydrated by consuming enough water throughout the day. For certain people, dehydration can be a migraine trigger.

4. A well-rounded diet

Ensure that your diet is well-balanced and that you eat frequent meals and snacks. Recognize and stay away from particular trigger foods, and think about getting individualized nutritional counsel from a trained dietitian.

5. Control Your Stress:

Use stress-reduction strategies including mindfulness, meditation, and deep breathing. Migraine prevention can be achieved with regular stress reduction techniques.

6. Frequent Workout:

Regularly partake in mild physical activities, such cycling, swimming, or walking. In addition to improving general wellbeing, exercise helps lessen migraine frequency.

7. Biofeedback:

A method called biofeedback aids people in regaining control over specific physiological processes. It can be helpful in preventing migraines and in managing stress.

8. Therapy based on cognitive behavior (CBT):

CBT is a type of psychotherapy that can assist people in recognizing and altering thought and behavior patterns associated with migraines. Reducing the frequency and intensity of episodes might be a successful outcome.

9. Control of Hormones:

Hormonal therapy may be taken into consideration for women whose migraines are impacted by fluctuations in their hormone levels. Hormone replacement therapy, hormonal contraception, and other hormonal therapies may be used in this situation.

10. Drugs for Preventive Care:

Certain drugs may be prescribed by medical professionals to avoid migraines. These could consist of:

Beta-blockers: Propranolol, for example.

Antidepressants: selective serotonin reuptake inhibitors (SSRIs) or tricyclic antidepressants.

Anti-seizure drugs: Valproic acid or topiramate, for example.

11. Neuromodulation Tools:

Non-pharmacological neuromodulation techniques, such as external trigeminal nerve stimulation (eTNS) or transcutaneous electrical nerve stimulation (TENS), may be employed to avoid migraines.

12. Botox injections:

As a preventative measure, people with chronic migraines (15 or more headache days per month) may benefit from botulinum toxin (Botox) injections.

13. Keep Your Lifestyle Consistent:

Develop and uphold regular eating, sleeping, and exercise schedules as well as consistent lifestyle practices. For certain people, migraines can be brought on by abrupt changes in their routine.

14. Observe and Modify:

Consistently assess the success of preventive measures and be prepared to modify the treatment plan after consulting with medical professionals. Finding the best combination of therapies may take some time.

It is advised that migraine sufferers collaborate closely with their medical professionals to create a customized preventive plan that takes into account their unique requirements and preferences. Optimizing migraine preventive measures requires regular follow-up consultations and open communication.

Conclusion

In conclusion, millions of people worldwide are impacted by migraines, which are intricate neurological conditions that go beyond simple headaches. Migraines are characterized by excruciating pain and frequently accompanying symptoms including nausea, light and sound sensitivity, and in rare cases, visual problems. Migraines have a major influence on the lives of those who suffer them.

Migraines are complex conditions resulting from a confluence of neurological, environmental, and hereditary variables. Though individual triggers might differ greatly, stress, hormone fluctuations, specific meals, and environmental variables are frequently identified as culprits. The cornerstones of migraine therapy include the identification and control of triggers as well as the application of acute and preventive medications.

Maintaining a healthy lifestyle, which includes regular sleep patterns, stress reduction, staying hydrated, and eating a balanced diet, is essential for managing migraines. The goal of preventive methods, which might include medicine and neuromodulation devices, is to lessen the frequency and intensity of migraine attacks.

Support networks and coping mechanisms are essential for overcoming the difficulties that migraines present. Creating a supportive environment, educating people, and understanding the condition all help to make managing this chronic illness more robust.

It is hoped that as science and medicine progress, migraine sufferers' quality of life will be enhanced, treatment methods will be improved, and awareness will be raised to lessen the stigma attached to this frequently crippling ailment.

Through the development of cooperative relationships among patients, medical professionals, and the community at large, the experience of living with migraines can be viewed with compassion, understanding, and a dedication to improving general health.

THE END